Symptoms	Type
Dull, aching pain on both sides of the head A feeling of pressure behind the eyes The sensation of tightness at the back of the head Tender neck or shoulder muscles	Tension
Sudden pain in the temples, the top of the head or behind your ears Tenderness or swelling to the top, sides, front or back of the head A sore scalp Jaw pain, typically when chewing or talking Visual problems, fatique, fever	Giant Cell Arteritis
Stabbing or burning pain centred over one eye or temple Severe or excruciating pain lasting from a few minutes to a few hours A red and watering eye A drooping or swollen eyelid A blocked or runny nose A shrunken or constricted pupil Sweating	Cluster
Throbbing pain in the forehead or cheeks Facial tenderness or swelling A blocked or runny nose Green or yellow discharge from the nose Earache Fever	Sinus
Throbbing pain on one side of the head Moderate to severe pain Blurred vision, seeing flashing lights or zigzag lines Increased sensitivity to light, smells or loud noises Feeling lightheaded Nausea and/or vomiting	Migraine

EXAMPLE

TIME

	begin	end	duration		begin	end	duration
1	10:30	12:30	2 hrs	3	19:30		
2	15:10	15:30	20 m	4			

LOCATION

tension	gca	cluster	sinus	migraine	neck
1		2 3			

SEVERITY

1	2	3	4	5	6	7 ✓	8	9	10

MILD — SEVERE

TRIGGERS

- [ ] coffee
- [ ] alcohol
- [ ] medication
- [ ] food
- [ ] weather
- [x] allergies
- [ ] insomnia
- [ ] stress
- [ ] bright light
- [ ] pc/tv screen
- [ ] reading
- [ ] noise
- [ ] eye strain
- [ ] sickness
- [ ] travel
- [x] motion
- [ ] anxiety
- [ ] pms
- [ ] smell

RELIEF MEASURES

medication	Took 2 painkillers 10 am + 3 pm
sleep/rest	
exercise	Neck massage helped relief pain
Other	

<table>
<tr><td></td><td>DATE</td><td></td></tr>
</table>

TIME

	begin	end	duration		begin	end	duration
1				3			
2				4			

LOCATION

tension	gca	cluster	sinus	migraine	neck

SEVERITY

1	2	3	4	5	6	7	8	9	10

MILD   SEVERE

TRIGGERS

☐ coffee	☐ insomnia	☐ eye strain	☐ smell
☐ alcohol	☐ stress	☐ sickness	☐
☐ medication	☐ bright light	☐ travel	☐
☐ food	☐ pc/tv screen	☐ motion	☐
☐ weather	☐ reading	☐ anxiety	☐
☐ allergies	☐ noise	☐ pms	☐

RELIEF MEASURES

medication

sleep/rest

exercise

Other

<table>
<tr><td></td><td></td><td></td><td></td><td>DATE</td><td></td></tr>
</table>

TIME

	begin	end	duration		begin	end	duration
1				3			
2				4			

LOCATION

tension	gca	cluster	sinus	migraine	neck

SEVERITY

1	2	3	4	5	6	7	8	9	10

MILD — SEVERE

TRIGGERS

☐ coffee	☐ insomnia	☐ eye strain	☐ smell
☐ alcohol	☐ stress	☐ sickness	☐
☐ medication	☐ bright light	☐ travel	☐
☐ food	☐ pc/tv screen	☐ motion	☐
☐ weather	☐ reading	☐ anxiety	☐
☐ allergies	☐ noise	☐ pms	☐

RELIEF MEASURES

medication	
sleep/rest	
exercise	
Other	

<table>
<tr><td colspan="7" align="center">DATE</td></tr>
</table>

TIME

	begin	end	duration		begin	end	duration
1				3			
2				4			

LOCATION

tension	gca	cluster	sinus	migraine	neck

SEVERITY

1	2	3	4	5	6	7	8	9	10

MILD   SEVERE

TRIGGERS

coffee	insomnia	eye strain	smell
alcohol	stress	sickness	
medication	bright light	travel	
food	pc/tv screen	motion	
weather	reading	anxiety	
allergies	noise	pms	

RELIEF MEASURES

medication

sleep/rest

exercise

Other

<table>
<tr><td></td><td></td><td></td><td></td><td style="background:#888;color:#fff">DATE</td><td></td><td></td><td></td></tr>
</table>

TIME

	begin	end	duration		begin	end	duration
1				3			
2				4			

LOCATION

tension	gca	cluster	sinus	migraine	neck

SEVERITY

1	2	3	4	5	6	7	8	9	10

MILD   SEVERE

TRIGGERS

☐ coffee	☐ insomnia	☐ eye strain	☐ smell
☐ alcohol	☐ stress	☐ sickness	☐
☐ medication	☐ bright light	☐ travel	☐
☐ food	☐ pc/tv screen	☐ motion	☐
☐ weather	☐ reading	☐ anxiety	☐
☐ allergies	☐ noise	☐ pms	☐

RELIEF MEASURES

medication	
sleep/rest	
exercise	
Other	

<table>
<tr><td colspan="7" align="center">DATE</td></tr>
</table>

TIME

	begin	end	duration		begin	end	duration
1				3			
2				4			

LOCATION

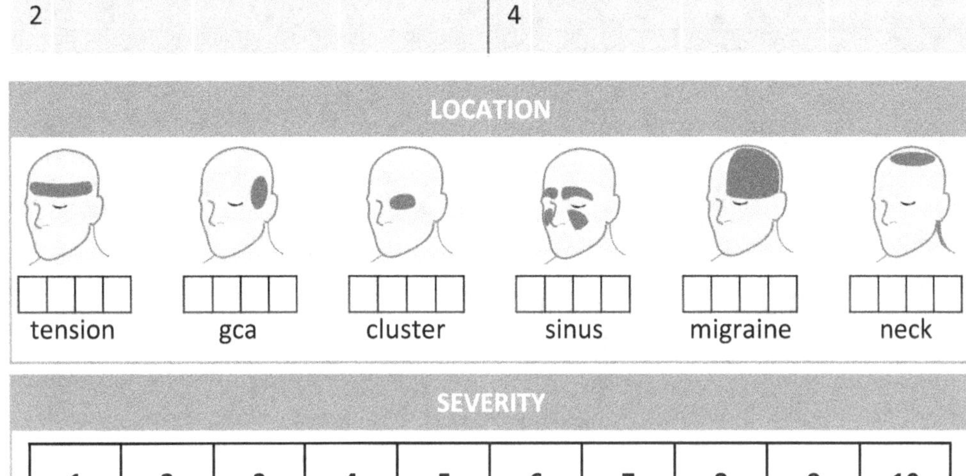

SEVERITY

1	2	3	4	5	6	7	8	9	10

MILD   SEVERE

TRIGGERS

☐ coffee	☐ insomnia	☐ eye strain	☐ smell
☐ alcohol	☐ stress	☐ sickness	☐
☐ medication	☐ bright light	☐ travel	☐
☐ food	☐ pc/tv screen	☐ motion	☐
☐ weather	☐ reading	☐ anxiety	☐
☐ allergies	☐ noise	☐ pms	☐

RELIEF MEASURES

medication

sleep/rest

exercise

Other

TIME

	begin	end	duration		begin	end	duration
1				3			
2				4			

LOCATION

tension   gca   cluster   sinus   migraine   neck

SEVERITY

1	2	3	4	5	6	7	8	9	10

MILD   SEVERE

TRIGGERS

- coffee
- alcohol
- medication
- food
- weather
- allergies
- insomnia
- stress
- bright light
- pc/tv screen
- reading
- noise
- eye strain
- sickness
- travel
- motion
- anxiety
- pms
- smell

RELIEF MEASURES

medication

sleep/rest

exercise

Other

<table>
<tr><td colspan="6" align="center">DATE</td></tr>
</table>

TIME

	begin	end	duration		begin	end	duration
1				3			
2				4			

LOCATION

tension	gca	cluster	sinus	migraine	neck

SEVERITY

1	2	3	4	5	6	7	8	9	10

MILD   SEVERE

TRIGGERS

☐ coffee	☐ insomnia	☐ eye strain	☐ smell
☐ alcohol	☐ stress	☐ sickness	☐
☐ medication	☐ bright light	☐ travel	☐
☐ food	☐ pc/tv screen	☐ motion	☐
☐ weather	☐ reading	☐ anxiety	☐
☐ allergies	☐ noise	☐ pms	☐

RELIEF MEASURES

medication

sleep/rest

exercise

Other

<table>
<tr><td></td><td>DATE</td><td></td></tr>
</table>

TIME

	begin	end	duration		begin	end	duration
1				3			
2				4			

LOCATION

tension	gca	cluster	sinus	migraine	neck

SEVERITY

1	2	3	4	5	6	7	8	9	10

MILD   SEVERE

TRIGGERS

☐ coffee	☐ insomnia	☐ eye strain	☐ smell
☐ alcohol	☐ stress	☐ sickness	☐
☐ medication	☐ bright light	☐ travel	☐
☐ food	☐ pc/tv screen	☐ motion	☐
☐ weather	☐ reading	☐ anxiety	☐
☐ allergies	☐ noise	☐ pms	☐

RELIEF MEASURES

medication

sleep/rest

exercise

Other

<table>
<tr><td colspan="7" align="center">DATE</td></tr>
</table>

TIME

	begin	end	duration		begin	end	duration
1				3			
2				4			

LOCATION

tension	gca	cluster	sinus	migraine	neck

SEVERITY

1	2	3	4	5	6	7	8	9	10

MILD   SEVERE

TRIGGERS

- [ ] coffee
- [ ] alcohol
- [ ] medication
- [ ] food
- [ ] weather
- [ ] allergies
- [ ] insomnia
- [ ] stress
- [ ] bright light
- [ ] pc/tv screen
- [ ] reading
- [ ] noise
- [ ] eye strain
- [ ] sickness
- [ ] travel
- [ ] motion
- [ ] anxiety
- [ ] pms
- [ ] smell

RELIEF MEASURES

medication

sleep/rest

exercise

Other

TIME

	begin	end	duration		begin	end	duration
1				3			
2				4			

LOCATION

tension   gca   cluster   sinus   migraine   neck

SEVERITY

1	2	3	4	5	6	7	8	9	10

MILD   SEVERE

TRIGGERS

- [ ] coffee
- [ ] alcohol
- [ ] medication
- [ ] food
- [ ] weather
- [ ] allergies
- [ ] insomnia
- [ ] stress
- [ ] bright light
- [ ] pc/tv screen
- [ ] reading
- [ ] noise
- [ ] eye strain
- [ ] sickness
- [ ] travel
- [ ] motion
- [ ] anxiety
- [ ] pms
- [ ] smell

RELIEF MEASURES

medication

sleep/rest

exercise

Other

TIME

	begin	end	duration		begin	end	duration
1				3			
2				4			

LOCATION

tension	gca	cluster	sinus	migraine	neck

SEVERITY

1	2	3	4	5	6	7	8	9	10

MILD — SEVERE

TRIGGERS

- ☐ coffee
- ☐ alcohol
- ☐ medication
- ☐ food
- ☐ weather
- ☐ allergies
- ☐ insomnia
- ☐ stress
- ☐ bright light
- ☐ pc/tv screen
- ☐ reading
- ☐ noise
- ☐ eye strain
- ☐ sickness
- ☐ travel
- ☐ motion
- ☐ anxiety
- ☐ pms
- ☐ smell

RELIEF MEASURES

medication

sleep/rest

exercise

Other

<table>
<tr><td colspan="7" align="center">DATE</td></tr>
</table>

<table>
<tr><td colspan="7" align="center">TIME</td></tr>
<tr><td></td><td>begin</td><td>end</td><td>duration</td><td>begin</td><td>end</td><td>duration</td></tr>
<tr><td>1</td><td></td><td></td><td></td><td>3</td><td></td><td></td></tr>
<tr><td>2</td><td></td><td></td><td></td><td>4</td><td></td><td></td></tr>
</table>

LOCATION

tension	gca	cluster	sinus	migraine	neck

SEVERITY

1	2	3	4	5	6	7	8	9	10

MILD   SEVERE

TRIGGERS

☐ coffee	☐ insomnia	☐ eye strain	☐ smell
☐ alcohol	☐ stress	☐ sickness	☐
☐ medication	☐ bright light	☐ travel	☐
☐ food	☐ pc/tv screen	☐ motion	☐
☐ weather	☐ reading	☐ anxiety	☐
☐ allergies	☐ noise	☐ pms	☐

RELIEF MEASURES

medication

sleep/rest

exercise

Other

<table>
<tr><td></td><td></td><td></td><td></td><td>**DATE**</td><td></td></tr>
</table>

TIME

	begin	end	duration		begin	end	duration
1				3			
2				4			

LOCATION

tension	gca	cluster	sinus	migraine	neck

SEVERITY

1	2	3	4	5	6	7	8	9	10

MILD   SEVERE

TRIGGERS

- [ ] coffee
- [ ] alcohol
- [ ] medication
- [ ] food
- [ ] weather
- [ ] allergies
- [ ] insomnia
- [ ] stress
- [ ] bright light
- [ ] pc/tv screen
- [ ] reading
- [ ] noise
- [ ] eye strain
- [ ] sickness
- [ ] travel
- [ ] motion
- [ ] anxiety
- [ ] pms
- [ ] smell

RELIEF MEASURES

medication

sleep/rest

exercise

Other

<table>
<tr><td></td><td>DATE</td><td></td></tr>
</table>

TIME

	begin	end	duration		begin	end	duration
1				3			
2				4			

LOCATION

tension	gca	cluster	sinus	migraine	neck

SEVERITY

1	2	3	4	5	6	7	8	9	10

MILD   SEVERE

TRIGGERS

☐ coffee	☐ insomnia	☐ eye strain	☐ smell
☐ alcohol	☐ stress	☐ sickness	☐
☐ medication	☐ bright light	☐ travel	☐
☐ food	☐ pc/tv screen	☐ motion	☐
☐ weather	☐ reading	☐ anxiety	☐
☐ allergies	☐ noise	☐ pms	☐

RELIEF MEASURES

medication

sleep/rest

exercise

Other

<table>
<tr><td colspan="7" align="center">**DATE**</td></tr>
</table>

TIME

	begin	end	duration		begin	end	duration
1				3			
2				4			

LOCATION

tension	gca	cluster	sinus	migraine	neck

SEVERITY

1	2	3	4	5	6	7	8	9	10

MILD · SEVERE

TRIGGERS

☐ coffee	☐ insomnia	☐ eye strain	☐ smell
☐ alcohol	☐ stress	☐ sickness	☐
☐ medication	☐ bright light	☐ travel	☐
☐ food	☐ pc/tv screen	☐ motion	☐
☐ weather	☐ reading	☐ anxiety	☐
☐ allergies	☐ noise	☐ pms	☐

RELIEF MEASURES

medication

sleep/rest

exercise

Other

<table>
<tr><td colspan="7" align="center">DATE</td></tr>
</table>

TIME

	begin	end	duration		begin	end	duration
1				3			
2				4			

LOCATION

tension	gca	cluster	sinus	migraine	neck
☐☐☐☐	☐☐☐☐	☐☐☐☐	☐☐☐☐	☐☐☐☐	☐☐☐☐

SEVERITY

1	2	3	4	5	6	7	8	9	10

MILD   SEVERE

TRIGGERS

☐ coffee	☐ insomnia	☐ eye strain	☐ smell
☐ alcohol	☐ stress	☐ sickness	☐
☐ medication	☐ bright light	☐ travel	☐
☐ food	☐ pc/tv screen	☐ motion	☐
☐ weather	☐ reading	☐ anxiety	☐
☐ allergies	☐ noise	☐ pms	☐

RELIEF MEASURES

medication	
sleep/rest	
exercise	
Other	

<table>
<tr><td colspan="7" align="center">DATE</td></tr>
</table>

TIME

	begin	end	duration		begin	end	duration
1				3			
2				4			

LOCATION

tension	gca	cluster	sinus	migraine	neck

SEVERITY

1	2	3	4	5	6	7	8	9	10

MILD — SEVERE

TRIGGERS

- [ ] coffee
- [ ] alcohol
- [ ] medication
- [ ] food
- [ ] weather
- [ ] allergies
- [ ] insomnia
- [ ] stress
- [ ] bright light
- [ ] pc/tv screen
- [ ] reading
- [ ] noise
- [ ] eye strain
- [ ] sickness
- [ ] travel
- [ ] motion
- [ ] anxiety
- [ ] pms
- [ ] smell

RELIEF MEASURES

medication	
sleep/rest	
exercise	
Other	

TIME

	begin	end	duration		begin	end	duration
1				3			
2				4			

LOCATION

tension	gca	cluster	sinus	migraine	neck

SEVERITY

1	2	3	4	5	6	7	8	9	10

MILD   SEVERE

TRIGGERS

- [ ] coffee
- [ ] alcohol
- [ ] medication
- [ ] food
- [ ] weather
- [ ] allergies
- [ ] insomnia
- [ ] stress
- [ ] bright light
- [ ] pc/tv screen
- [ ] reading
- [ ] noise
- [ ] eye strain
- [ ] sickness
- [ ] travel
- [ ] motion
- [ ] anxiety
- [ ] pms
- [ ] smell

RELIEF MEASURES

medication

sleep/rest

exercise

Other

<table>
<tr><td></td><td></td><td></td><td>DATE</td><td></td><td></td></tr>
</table>

TIME

	begin	end	duration		begin	end	duration
1				3			
2				4			

LOCATION

tension	gca	cluster	sinus	migraine	neck

SEVERITY

1	2	3	4	5	6	7	8	9	10

MILD   SEVERE

TRIGGERS

☐ coffee	☐ insomnia	☐ eye strain	☐ smell
☐ alcohol	☐ stress	☐ sickness	☐
☐ medication	☐ bright light	☐ travel	☐
☐ food	☐ pc/tv screen	☐ motion	☐
☐ weather	☐ reading	☐ anxiety	☐
☐ allergies	☐ noise	☐ pms	☐

RELIEF MEASURES

medication

sleep/rest

exercise

Other

<table>
<tr><td></td><td></td><td></td><td></td><td>DATE</td><td></td><td></td><td></td></tr>
</table>

TIME

	begin	end	duration		begin	end	duration
1				3			
2				4			

LOCATION

tension	gca	cluster	sinus	migraine	neck

SEVERITY

1	2	3	4	5	6	7	8	9	10

MILD   SEVERE

TRIGGERS

☐ coffee	☐ insomnia	☐ eye strain	☐ smell
☐ alcohol	☐ stress	☐ sickness	☐
☐ medication	☐ bright light	☐ travel	☐
☐ food	☐ pc/tv screen	☐ motion	☐
☐ weather	☐ reading	☐ anxiety	☐
☐ allergies	☐ noise	☐ pms	☐

RELIEF MEASURES

medication

sleep/rest

exercise

Other

<table>
<tr><td></td><td style="background:#999;color:#fff;text-align:center">DATE</td><td></td></tr>
</table>

TIME

	begin	end	duration		begin	end	duration
1				3			
2				4			

LOCATION

tension	gca	cluster	sinus	migraine	neck
▢▢▢▢	▢▢▢▢	▢▢▢▢	▢▢▢▢	▢▢▢▢	▢▢▢▢

SEVERITY

1	2	3	4	5	6	7	8	9	10

MILD   SEVERE

TRIGGERS

☐ coffee	☐ insomnia	☐ eye strain	☐ smell
☐ alcohol	☐ stress	☐ sickness	☐
☐ medication	☐ bright light	☐ travel	☐
☐ food	☐ pc/tv screen	☐ motion	☐
☐ weather	☐ reading	☐ anxiety	☐
☐ allergies	☐ noise	☐ pms	☐

RELIEF MEASURES

medication

sleep/rest

exercise

Other

<table>
<tr><td></td><td>DATE</td><td></td></tr>
</table>

TIME

	begin	end	duration		begin	end	duration
1				3			
2				4			

LOCATION

□□□□	□□□□	□□□□	□□□□	□□□□	□□□□
tension	gca	cluster	sinus	migraine	neck

SEVERITY

1	2	3	4	5	6	7	8	9	10

MILD   SEVERE

TRIGGERS

□ coffee	□ insomnia	□ eye strain	□ smell
□ alcohol	□ stress	□ sickness	□
□ medication	□ bright light	□ travel	□
□ food	□ pc/tv screen	□ motion	□
□ weather	□ reading	□ anxiety	□
□ allergies	□ noise	□ pms	□

RELIEF MEASURES

medication	
sleep/rest	
exercise	
Other	

<table>
<tr><td colspan="7" align="center">DATE</td></tr>
</table>

<table>
<tr><td colspan="6" align="center">TIME</td></tr>
<tr><td>begin</td><td>end</td><td>duration</td><td>begin</td><td>end</td><td>duration</td></tr>
<tr><td>1</td><td></td><td></td><td>3</td><td></td><td></td></tr>
<tr><td>2</td><td></td><td></td><td>4</td><td></td><td></td></tr>
</table>

<table>
<tr><td colspan="6" align="center">LOCATION</td></tr>
<tr><td>tension</td><td>gca</td><td>cluster</td><td>sinus</td><td>migraine</td><td>neck</td></tr>
</table>

<table>
<tr><td colspan="10" align="center">SEVERITY</td></tr>
<tr><td>1</td><td>2</td><td>3</td><td>4</td><td>5</td><td>6</td><td>7</td><td>8</td><td>9</td><td>10</td></tr>
</table>

MILD · SEVERE

<table>
<tr><td colspan="4" align="center">TRIGGERS</td></tr>
<tr><td>☐ coffee</td><td>☐ insomnia</td><td>☐ eye strain</td><td>☐ smell</td></tr>
<tr><td>☐ alcohol</td><td>☐ stress</td><td>☐ sickness</td><td>☐</td></tr>
<tr><td>☐ medication</td><td>☐ bright light</td><td>☐ travel</td><td>☐</td></tr>
<tr><td>☐ food</td><td>☐ pc/tv screen</td><td>☐ motion</td><td>☐</td></tr>
<tr><td>☐ weather</td><td>☐ reading</td><td>☐ anxiety</td><td>☐</td></tr>
<tr><td>☐ allergies</td><td>☐ noise</td><td>☐ pms</td><td>☐</td></tr>
</table>

<table>
<tr><td colspan="2" align="center">RELIEF MEASURES</td></tr>
<tr><td>medication</td><td></td></tr>
<tr><td>sleep/rest</td><td></td></tr>
<tr><td>exercise</td><td></td></tr>
<tr><td>Other</td><td></td></tr>
</table>

<table>
<tr><td></td><td></td><td colspan="7" align="center">DATE</td><td></td></tr>
</table>

TIME

	begin	end	duration		begin	end	duration
1				3			
2				4			

LOCATION

tension	gca	cluster	sinus	migraine	neck

SEVERITY

1	2	3	4	5	6	7	8	9	10

MILD — SEVERE

TRIGGERS

☐ coffee	☐ insomnia	☐ eye strain	☐ smell
☐ alcohol	☐ stress	☐ sickness	☐
☐ medication	☐ bright light	☐ travel	☐
☐ food	☐ pc/tv screen	☐ motion	☐
☐ weather	☐ reading	☐ anxiety	☐
☐ allergies	☐ noise	☐ pms	☐

RELIEF MEASURES

medication

sleep/rest

exercise

Other

<table>
<tr><td></td><td>DATE</td><td></td></tr>
</table>

TIME

	begin	end	duration		begin	end	duration
1				3			
2				4			

LOCATION

tension	gca	cluster	sinus	migraine	neck

SEVERITY

1	2	3	4	5	6	7	8	9	10

MILD   SEVERE

TRIGGERS

☐ coffee	☐ insomnia	☐ eye strain	☐ smell
☐ alcohol	☐ stress	☐ sickness	☐
☐ medication	☐ bright light	☐ travel	☐
☐ food	☐ pc/tv screen	☐ motion	☐
☐ weather	☐ reading	☐ anxiety	☐
☐ allergies	☐ noise	☐ pms	☐

RELIEF MEASURES

medication

sleep/rest

exercise

Other

<table>
<tr><td></td><td></td><td></td><td></td><td></td><td>DATE</td><td></td></tr>
</table>

TIME

	begin	end	duration		begin	end	duration
1				3			
2				4			

LOCATION

tension	gca	cluster	sinus	migraine	neck

SEVERITY

1	2	3	4	5	6	7	8	9	10

MILD — SEVERE

TRIGGERS

- coffee
- alcohol
- medication
- food
- weather
- allergies
- insomnia
- stress
- bright light
- pc/tv screen
- reading
- noise
- eye strain
- sickness
- travel
- motion
- anxiety
- pms
- smell

RELIEF MEASURES

medication

sleep/rest

exercise

Other

<table>
<tr><td></td><td>DATE</td><td></td></tr>
</table>

TIME

	begin	end	duration		begin	end	duration
1				3			
2				4			

LOCATION

tension	gca	cluster	sinus	migraine	neck

SEVERITY

1	2	3	4	5	6	7	8	9	10

MILD — SEVERE

TRIGGERS

☐ coffee	☐ insomnia	☐ eye strain	☐ smell
☐ alcohol	☐ stress	☐ sickness	☐
☐ medication	☐ bright light	☐ travel	☐
☐ food	☐ pc/tv screen	☐ motion	☐
☐ weather	☐ reading	☐ anxiety	☐
☐ allergies	☐ noise	☐ pms	☐

RELIEF MEASURES

medication

sleep/rest

exercise

Other

<table>
<tr><td></td><td></td><td></td><td></td><td></td><td>DATE</td><td></td><td></td></tr>
</table>

TIME

	begin	end	duration		begin	end	duration
1				3			
2				4			

LOCATION

tension	gca	cluster	sinus	migraine	neck

SEVERITY

1	2	3	4	5	6	7	8	9	10

MILD   SEVERE

TRIGGERS

☐ coffee	☐ insomnia	☐ eye strain	☐ smell
☐ alcohol	☐ stress	☐ sickness	☐
☐ medication	☐ bright light	☐ travel	☐
☐ food	☐ pc/tv screen	☐ motion	☐
☐ weather	☐ reading	☐ anxiety	☐
☐ allergies	☐ noise	☐ pms	☐

RELIEF MEASURES

medication	
sleep/rest	
exercise	
Other	

<table>
<tr><td colspan="7" align="center">DATE</td></tr>
</table>

TIME

	begin	end	duration		begin	end	duration
1				3			
2				4			

LOCATION

tension	gca	cluster	sinus	migraine	neck

SEVERITY

1	2	3	4	5	6	7	8	9	10

MILD · SEVERE

TRIGGERS

- [ ] coffee
- [ ] alcohol
- [ ] medication
- [ ] food
- [ ] weather
- [ ] allergies
- [ ] insomnia
- [ ] stress
- [ ] bright light
- [ ] pc/tv screen
- [ ] reading
- [ ] noise
- [ ] eye strain
- [ ] sickness
- [ ] travel
- [ ] motion
- [ ] anxiety
- [ ] pms
- [ ] smell
- [ ]
- [ ]
- [ ]
- [ ]
- [ ]

RELIEF MEASURES

medication

sleep/rest

exercise

Other

<table>
<tr><td></td><td>DATE</td><td></td></tr>
</table>

TIME

	begin	end	duration		begin	end	duration
1				3			
2				4			

LOCATION

tension	gca	cluster	sinus	migraine	neck

SEVERITY

1	2	3	4	5	6	7	8	9	10

MILD — SEVERE

TRIGGERS

☐ coffee	☐ insomnia	☐ eye strain	☐ smell
☐ alcohol	☐ stress	☐ sickness	☐
☐ medication	☐ bright light	☐ travel	☐
☐ food	☐ pc/tv screen	☐ motion	☐
☐ weather	☐ reading	☐ anxiety	☐
☐ allergies	☐ noise	☐ pms	☐

RELIEF MEASURES

medication

sleep/rest

exercise

Other

<table>
<tr><td></td><td>DATE</td><td></td></tr>
</table>

TIME

	begin	end	duration		begin	end	duration
1				3			
2				4			

LOCATION

tension	gca	cluster	sinus	migraine	neck

SEVERITY

1	2	3	4	5	6	7	8	9	10

MILD   SEVERE

TRIGGERS

☐ coffee	☐ insomnia	☐ eye strain	☐ smell
☐ alcohol	☐ stress	☐ sickness	☐
☐ medication	☐ bright light	☐ travel	☐
☐ food	☐ pc/tv screen	☐ motion	☐
☐ weather	☐ reading	☐ anxiety	☐
☐ allergies	☐ noise	☐ pms	☐

RELIEF MEASURES

medication	
sleep/rest	
exercise	
Other	

TIME

	begin	end	duration		begin	end	duration
1				3			
2				4			

LOCATION

tension   gca   cluster   sinus   migraine   neck

SEVERITY

1	2	3	4	5	6	7	8	9	10

MILD   SEVERE

TRIGGERS

- coffee
- alcohol
- medication
- food
- weather
- allergies
- insomnia
- stress
- bright light
- pc/tv screen
- reading
- noise
- eye strain
- sickness
- travel
- motion
- anxiety
- pms
- smell

RELIEF MEASURES

medication

sleep/rest

exercise

Other

DATE

TIME

	begin	end	duration		begin	end	duration
1				3			
2				4			

LOCATION

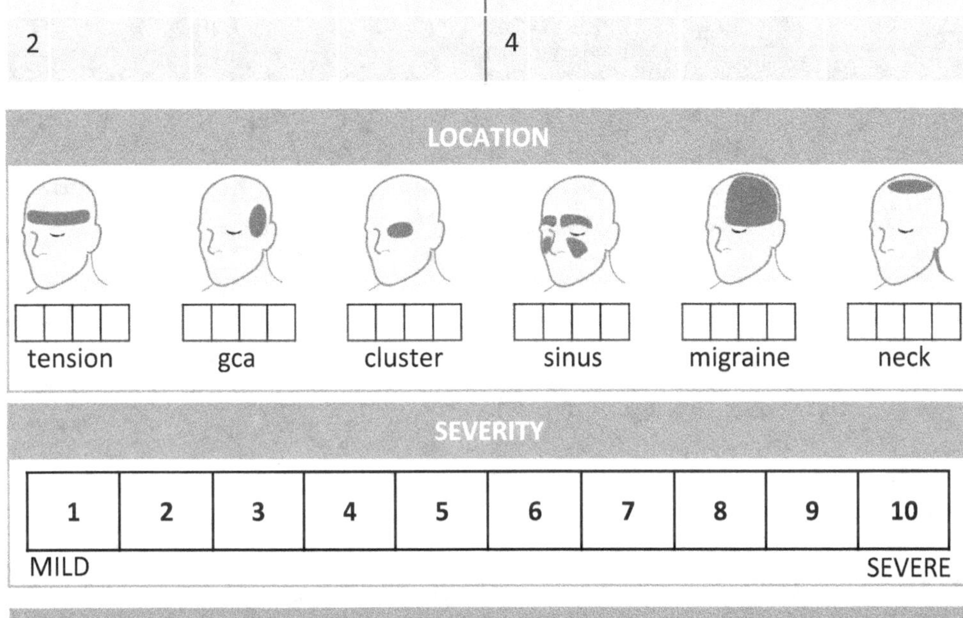

SEVERITY

1	2	3	4	5	6	7	8	9	10

MILD — SEVERE

TRIGGERS

☐ coffee	☐ insomnia	☐ eye strain	☐ smell
☐ alcohol	☐ stress	☐ sickness	☐
☐ medication	☐ bright light	☐ travel	☐
☐ food	☐ pc/tv screen	☐ motion	☐
☐ weather	☐ reading	☐ anxiety	☐
☐ allergies	☐ noise	☐ pms	☐

RELIEF MEASURES

medication

sleep/rest

exercise

Other

<table>
<tr><td></td><td></td><td></td><td></td><td></td><td>DATE</td><td></td></tr>
</table>

TIME

	begin	end	duration		begin	end	duration
1				3			
2				4			

LOCATION

tension	gca	cluster	sinus	migraine	neck

SEVERITY

1	2	3	4	5	6	7	8	9	10

MILD   SEVERE

TRIGGERS

☐ coffee	☐ insomnia	☐ eye strain	☐ smell
☐ alcohol	☐ stress	☐ sickness	☐
☐ medication	☐ bright light	☐ travel	☐
☐ food	☐ pc/tv screen	☐ motion	☐
☐ weather	☐ reading	☐ anxiety	☐
☐ allergies	☐ noise	☐ pms	☐

RELIEF MEASURES

medication

sleep/rest

exercise

Other

TIME

	begin	end	duration		begin	end	duration
1				3			
2				4			

LOCATION

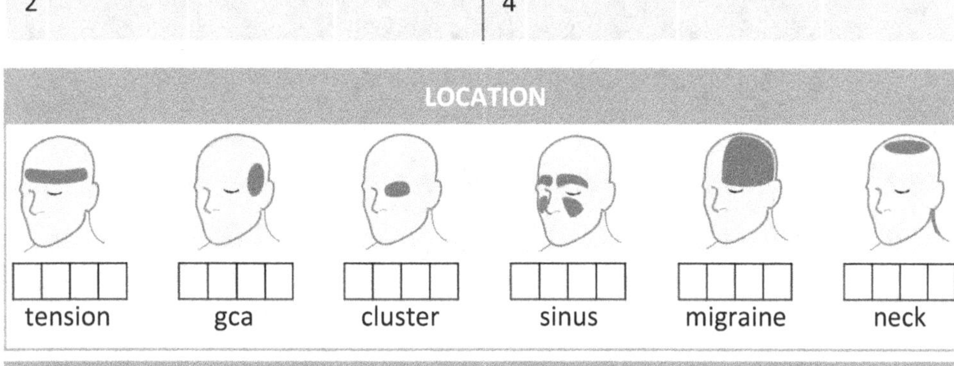

SEVERITY

1	2	3	4	5	6	7	8	9	10

MILD · SEVERE

TRIGGERS

- [ ] coffee
- [ ] alcohol
- [ ] medication
- [ ] food
- [ ] weather
- [ ] allergies
- [ ] insomnia
- [ ] stress
- [ ] bright light
- [ ] pc/tv screen
- [ ] reading
- [ ] noise
- [ ] eye strain
- [ ] sickness
- [ ] travel
- [ ] motion
- [ ] anxiety
- [ ] pms
- [ ] smell
- [ ]
- [ ]
- [ ]
- [ ]
- [ ]

RELIEF MEASURES

medication

sleep/rest

exercise

Other

DATE	

TIME

	begin	end	duration		begin	end	duration
1				3			
2				4			

LOCATION

tension	gca	cluster	sinus	migraine	neck

SEVERITY

1	2	3	4	5	6	7	8	9	10

MILD — SEVERE

TRIGGERS

- [ ] coffee
- [ ] alcohol
- [ ] medication
- [ ] food
- [ ] weather
- [ ] allergies
- [ ] insomnia
- [ ] stress
- [ ] bright light
- [ ] pc/tv screen
- [ ] reading
- [ ] noise
- [ ] eye strain
- [ ] sickness
- [ ] travel
- [ ] motion
- [ ] anxiety
- [ ] pms
- [ ] smell

RELIEF MEASURES

medication

sleep/rest

exercise

Other

<table>
<tr><td></td><td colspan="3" align="center">DATE</td><td></td></tr>
</table>

TIME

	begin	end	duration		begin	end	duration
1				3			
2				4			

LOCATION

tension	gca	cluster	sinus	migraine	neck
☐☐☐☐	☐☐☐☐	☐☐☐☐	☐☐☐☐	☐☐☐☐	☐☐☐☐

SEVERITY

1	2	3	4	5	6	7	8	9	10

MILD   SEVERE

TRIGGERS

☐ coffee	☐ insomnia	☐ eye strain	☐ smell
☐ alcohol	☐ stress	☐ sickness	☐
☐ medication	☐ bright light	☐ travel	☐
☐ food	☐ pc/tv screen	☐ motion	☐
☐ weather	☐ reading	☐ anxiety	☐
☐ allergies	☐ noise	☐ pms	☐

RELIEF MEASURES

medication

sleep/rest

exercise

Other

<table>
<tr><td colspan="7" align="center">DATE</td></tr>
</table>

TIME

	begin	end	duration		begin	end	duration
1				3			
2				4			

LOCATION

tension	gca	cluster	sinus	migraine	neck

SEVERITY

1	2	3	4	5	6	7	8	9	10

MILD — SEVERE

TRIGGERS

☐ coffee	☐ insomnia	☐ eye strain	☐ smell
☐ alcohol	☐ stress	☐ sickness	☐
☐ medication	☐ bright light	☐ travel	☐
☐ food	☐ pc/tv screen	☐ motion	☐
☐ weather	☐ reading	☐ anxiety	☐
☐ allergies	☐ noise	☐ pms	☐

RELIEF MEASURES

medication

sleep/rest

exercise

Other

<table>
<tr><td></td><td>DATE</td><td></td></tr>
</table>

TIME

	begin	end	duration		begin	end	duration
1				3			
2				4			

LOCATION

tension	gca	cluster	sinus	migraine	neck

SEVERITY

1	2	3	4	5	6	7	8	9	10

MILD   SEVERE

TRIGGERS

☐ coffee	☐ insomnia	☐ eye strain	☐ smell
☐ alcohol	☐ stress	☐ sickness	☐
☐ medication	☐ bright light	☐ travel	☐
☐ food	☐ pc/tv screen	☐ motion	☐
☐ weather	☐ reading	☐ anxiety	☐
☐ allergies	☐ noise	☐ pms	☐

RELIEF MEASURES

medication

sleep/rest

exercise

Other

<table>
<tr><td></td><td></td><td></td><td></td><td>DATE</td><td></td><td></td><td></td></tr>
</table>

TIME

	begin	end	duration		begin	end	duration
1				**3**			
2				**4**			

LOCATION

tension	gca	cluster	sinus	migraine	neck

SEVERITY

1	2	3	4	5	6	7	8	9	10

MILD   SEVERE

TRIGGERS

- ☐ coffee
- ☐ alcohol
- ☐ medication
- ☐ food
- ☐ weather
- ☐ allergies
- ☐ insomnia
- ☐ stress
- ☐ bright light
- ☐ pc/tv screen
- ☐ reading
- ☐ noise
- ☐ eye strain
- ☐ sickness
- ☐ travel
- ☐ motion
- ☐ anxiety
- ☐ pms
- ☐ smell
- ☐
- ☐
- ☐
- ☐
- ☐

RELIEF MEASURES

medication	
sleep/rest	
exercise	
Other	

<table>
<tr><td></td><td colspan="3" style="text-align:center">DATE</td><td></td></tr>
</table>

TIME

	begin	end	duration		begin	end	duration
1				3			
2				4			

LOCATION

tension	gca	cluster	sinus	migraine	neck

SEVERITY

1	2	3	4	5	6	7	8	9	10

MILD — SEVERE

TRIGGERS

☐ coffee	☐ insomnia	☐ eye strain	☐ smell
☐ alcohol	☐ stress	☐ sickness	☐
☐ medication	☐ bright light	☐ travel	☐
☐ food	☐ pc/tv screen	☐ motion	☐
☐ weather	☐ reading	☐ anxiety	☐
☐ allergies	☐ noise	☐ pms	☐

RELIEF MEASURES

medication

sleep/rest

exercise

Other

<table>
<tr><td></td><td>DATE</td><td></td></tr>
</table>

TIME

	begin	end	duration		begin	end	duration
1				3			
2				4			

LOCATION

tension	gca	cluster	sinus	migraine	neck

SEVERITY

1	2	3	4	5	6	7	8	9	10

MILD — SEVERE

TRIGGERS

☐ coffee	☐ insomnia	☐ eye strain	☐ smell
☐ alcohol	☐ stress	☐ sickness	☐
☐ medication	☐ bright light	☐ travel	☐
☐ food	☐ pc/tv screen	☐ motion	☐
☐ weather	☐ reading	☐ anxiety	☐
☐ allergies	☐ noise	☐ pms	☐

RELIEF MEASURES

medication

sleep/rest

exercise

Other

DATE	

TIME

	begin	end	duration		begin	end	duration
1				3			
2				4			

LOCATION

tension	gca	cluster	sinus	migraine	neck
☐☐☐☐	☐☐☐☐	☐☐☐☐	☐☐☐☐	☐☐☐☐	☐☐☐☐

SEVERITY

1	2	3	4	5	6	7	8	9	10

MILD ... SEVERE

TRIGGERS

☐ coffee	☐ insomnia	☐ eye strain	☐ smell
☐ alcohol	☐ stress	☐ sickness	☐
☐ medication	☐ bright light	☐ travel	☐
☐ food	☐ pc/tv screen	☐ motion	☐
☐ weather	☐ reading	☐ anxiety	☐
☐ allergies	☐ noise	☐ pms	☐

RELIEF MEASURES

medication

sleep/rest

exercise

Other

<table>
<tr><td></td><td>**DATE**</td><td></td></tr>
</table>

TIME

	begin	end	duration		begin	end	duration
1				3			
2				4			

LOCATION

tension	gca	cluster	sinus	migraine	neck

SEVERITY

1	2	3	4	5	6	7	8	9	10

MILD　　　　　　　　　　　　　　　　　　　　　　　　　SEVERE

TRIGGERS

☐ coffee	☐ insomnia	☐ eye strain	☐ smell
☐ alcohol	☐ stress	☐ sickness	☐
☐ medication	☐ bright light	☐ travel	☐
☐ food	☐ pc/tv screen	☐ motion	☐
☐ weather	☐ reading	☐ anxiety	☐
☐ allergies	☐ noise	☐ pms	☐

RELIEF MEASURES

medication

sleep/rest

exercise

Other

<table>
<tr><td></td><td colspan="3">DATE</td><td></td></tr>
</table>

TIME

	begin	end	duration		begin	end	duration
1				3			
2				4			

LOCATION

tension	gca	cluster	sinus	migraine	neck
☐☐☐☐	☐☐☐☐	☐☐☐☐	☐☐☐☐	☐☐☐☐	☐☐☐☐

SEVERITY

1	2	3	4	5	6	7	8	9	10

MILD   SEVERE

TRIGGERS

☐ coffee	☐ insomnia	☐ eye strain	☐ smell
☐ alcohol	☐ stress	☐ sickness	☐
☐ medication	☐ bright light	☐ travel	☐
☐ food	☐ pc/tv screen	☐ motion	☐
☐ weather	☐ reading	☐ anxiety	☐
☐ allergies	☐ noise	☐ pms	☐

RELIEF MEASURES

medication

sleep/rest

exercise

Other

TIME

	begin	end	duration		begin	end	duration
1				3			
2				4			

LOCATION

tension	gca	cluster	sinus	migraine	neck

SEVERITY

1	2	3	4	5	6	7	8	9	10

MILD   SEVERE

TRIGGERS

☐ coffee	☐ insomnia	☐ eye strain	☐ smell
☐ alcohol	☐ stress	☐ sickness	☐
☐ medication	☐ bright light	☐ travel	☐
☐ food	☐ pc/tv screen	☐ motion	☐
☐ weather	☐ reading	☐ anxiety	☐
☐ allergies	☐ noise	☐ pms	☐

RELIEF MEASURES

medication

sleep/rest

exercise

Other

<table>
<tr><td></td><td style="background:#888;color:white;text-align:center">DATE</td><td></td></tr>
</table>

<table><tr><td colspan="7" style="text-align:center">TIME</td></tr></table>

	begin	end	duration		begin	end	duration
1				3			
2				4			

LOCATION

tension	gca	cluster	sinus	migraine	neck

SEVERITY

1	2	3	4	5	6	7	8	9	10

MILD   SEVERE

TRIGGERS

☐ coffee	☐ insomnia	☐ eye strain	☐ smell
☐ alcohol	☐ stress	☐ sickness	☐
☐ medication	☐ bright light	☐ travel	☐
☐ food	☐ pc/tv screen	☐ motion	☐
☐ weather	☐ reading	☐ anxiety	☐
☐ allergies	☐ noise	☐ pms	☐

RELIEF MEASURES

medication

sleep/rest

exercise

Other

TIME

	begin	end	duration		begin	end	duration
1				3			
2				4			

LOCATION

tension	gca	cluster	sinus	migraine	neck

SEVERITY

1	2	3	4	5	6	7	8	9	10

MILD — SEVERE

TRIGGERS

- ☐ coffee
- ☐ alcohol
- ☐ medication
- ☐ food
- ☐ weather
- ☐ allergies
- ☐ insomnia
- ☐ stress
- ☐ bright light
- ☐ pc/tv screen
- ☐ reading
- ☐ noise
- ☐ eye strain
- ☐ sickness
- ☐ travel
- ☐ motion
- ☐ anxiety
- ☐ pms
- ☐ smell

RELIEF MEASURES

medication

sleep/rest

exercise

Other

<table>
<tr><td></td><td colspan="6" align="center">DATE</td></tr>
</table>

TIME

	begin	end	duration		begin	end	duration
1				3			
2				4			

LOCATION

tension	gca	cluster	sinus	migraine	neck

SEVERITY

1	2	3	4	5	6	7	8	9	10

MILD — SEVERE

TRIGGERS

- [ ] coffee
- [ ] alcohol
- [ ] medication
- [ ] food
- [ ] weather
- [ ] allergies
- [ ] insomnia
- [ ] stress
- [ ] bright light
- [ ] pc/tv screen
- [ ] reading
- [ ] noise
- [ ] eye strain
- [ ] sickness
- [ ] travel
- [ ] motion
- [ ] anxiety
- [ ] pms
- [ ] smell

RELIEF MEASURES

medication

sleep/rest

exercise

Other

<table>
<tr><td></td><td colspan="6">DATE</td></tr>
</table>

TIME

	begin	end	duration		begin	end	duration
1				3			
2				4			

LOCATION

tension	gca	cluster	sinus	migraine	neck

SEVERITY

1	2	3	4	5	6	7	8	9	10

MILD   SEVERE

TRIGGERS

☐ coffee	☐ insomnia	☐ eye strain	☐ smell
☐ alcohol	☐ stress	☐ sickness	☐
☐ medication	☐ bright light	☐ travel	☐
☐ food	☐ pc/tv screen	☐ motion	☐
☐ weather	☐ reading	☐ anxiety	☐
☐ allergies	☐ noise	☐ pms	☐

RELIEF MEASURES

medication

sleep/rest

exercise

Other

<table>
<tr><td colspan="7" align="center">DATE</td></tr>
</table>

TIME

	begin	end	duration		begin	end	duration
1				3			
2				4			

LOCATION

tension	gca	cluster	sinus	migraine	neck

SEVERITY

1	2	3	4	5	6	7	8	9	10

MILD   SEVERE

TRIGGERS

- ☐ coffee
- ☐ alcohol
- ☐ medication
- ☐ food
- ☐ weather
- ☐ allergies
- ☐ insomnia
- ☐ stress
- ☐ bright light
- ☐ pc/tv screen
- ☐ reading
- ☐ noise
- ☐ eye strain
- ☐ sickness
- ☐ travel
- ☐ motion
- ☐ anxiety
- ☐ pms
- ☐ smell
- ☐
- ☐
- ☐
- ☐
- ☐

RELIEF MEASURES

medication

sleep/rest

exercise

Other

<table>
<tr><td></td><td align="right">DATE</td><td></td></tr>
</table>

TIME

	begin	end	duration		begin	end	duration
1				3			
2				4			

LOCATION

tension	gca	cluster	sinus	migraine	neck

SEVERITY

1	2	3	4	5	6	7	8	9	10

MILD ... SEVERE

TRIGGERS

☐ coffee	☐ insomnia	☐ eye strain	☐ smell
☐ alcohol	☐ stress	☐ sickness	☐
☐ medication	☐ bright light	☐ travel	☐
☐ food	☐ pc/tv screen	☐ motion	☐
☐ weather	☐ reading	☐ anxiety	☐
☐ allergies	☐ noise	☐ pms	☐

RELIEF MEASURES

medication

sleep/rest

exercise

Other

<table>
<tr><td colspan="7" align="center">DATE</td></tr>
</table>

	begin	end	duration		begin	end	duration
TIME							
1				3			
2				4			

LOCATION

tension	gca	cluster	sinus	migraine	neck

SEVERITY

1	2	3	4	5	6	7	8	9	10

MILD   SEVERE

TRIGGERS

☐ coffee	☐ insomnia	☐ eye strain	☐ smell
☐ alcohol	☐ stress	☐ sickness	☐
☐ medication	☐ bright light	☐ travel	☐
☐ food	☐ pc/tv screen	☐ motion	☐
☐ weather	☐ reading	☐ anxiety	☐
☐ allergies	☐ noise	☐ pms	☐

RELIEF MEASURES

medication

sleep/rest

exercise

Other

<table>
<tr><td></td><td></td><td></td><td style="background:#999;color:#fff;text-align:center">DATE</td><td></td><td></td><td></td></tr>
</table>

TIME

	begin	end	duration		begin	end	duration
1				**3**			
2				**4**			

LOCATION

☐☐☐☐	☐☐☐☐	☐☐☐☐	☐☐☐☐	☐☐☐☐	☐☐☐☐
tension	gca	cluster	sinus	migraine	neck

SEVERITY

1	2	3	4	5	6	7	8	9	10

MILD   SEVERE

TRIGGERS

☐ coffee	☐ insomnia	☐ eye strain	☐ smell
☐ alcohol	☐ stress	☐ sickness	☐
☐ medication	☐ bright light	☐ travel	☐
☐ food	☐ pc/tv screen	☐ motion	☐
☐ weather	☐ reading	☐ anxiety	☐
☐ allergies	☐ noise	☐ pms	☐

RELIEF MEASURES

medication

sleep/rest

exercise

Other

	begin	end	duration		begin	end	duration
1				3			
2				4			

tension	gca	cluster	sinus	migraine	neck

1	2	3	4	5	6	7	8	9	10

MILD   SEVERE

- ☐ coffee
- ☐ alcohol
- ☐ medication
- ☐ food
- ☐ weather
- ☐ allergies
- ☐ insomnia
- ☐ stress
- ☐ bright light
- ☐ pc/tv screen
- ☐ reading
- ☐ noise
- ☐ eye strain
- ☐ sickness
- ☐ travel
- ☐ motion
- ☐ anxiety
- ☐ pms
- ☐ smell
- ☐
- ☐
- ☐
- ☐
- ☐

medication

sleep/rest

exercise

Other

<table>
<tr><td></td><td></td><td></td><td></td><td>DATE</td><td></td></tr>
</table>

TIME

	begin	end	duration		begin	end	duration
1				3			
2				4			

LOCATION

☐☐☐☐	☐☐☐☐	☐☐☐☐	☐☐☐☐	☐☐☐☐	☐☐☐☐
tension	gca	cluster	sinus	migraine	neck

SEVERITY

1	2	3	4	5	6	7	8	9	10

MILD   SEVERE

TRIGGERS

☐ coffee	☐ insomnia	☐ eye strain	☐ smell
☐ alcohol	☐ stress	☐ sickness	☐
☐ medication	☐ bright light	☐ travel	☐
☐ food	☐ pc/tv screen	☐ motion	☐
☐ weather	☐ reading	☐ anxiety	☐
☐ allergies	☐ noise	☐ pms	☐

RELIEF MEASURES

medication	
sleep/rest	
exercise	
Other	

TIME

	begin	end	duration		begin	end	duration
1				3			
2				4			

LOCATION

tension	gca	cluster	sinus	migraine	neck

SEVERITY

1	2	3	4	5	6	7	8	9	10

MILD   SEVERE

TRIGGERS

- ☐ coffee
- ☐ alcohol
- ☐ medication
- ☐ food
- ☐ weather
- ☐ allergies
- ☐ insomnia
- ☐ stress
- ☐ bright light
- ☐ pc/tv screen
- ☐ reading
- ☐ noise
- ☐ eye strain
- ☐ sickness
- ☐ travel
- ☐ motion
- ☐ anxiety
- ☐ pms
- ☐ smell

RELIEF MEASURES

medication

sleep/rest

exercise

Other

TIME

	begin	end	duration		begin	end	duration
1				3			
2				4			

LOCATION

tension   gca   cluster   sinus   migraine   neck

SEVERITY

1	2	3	4	5	6	7	8	9	10

MILD   SEVERE

TRIGGERS

☐ coffee	☐ insomnia	☐ eye strain	☐ smell
☐ alcohol	☐ stress	☐ sickness	☐
☐ medication	☐ bright light	☐ travel	☐
☐ food	☐ pc/tv screen	☐ motion	☐
☐ weather	☐ reading	☐ anxiety	☐
☐ allergies	☐ noise	☐ pms	☐

RELIEF MEASURES

medication

sleep/rest

exercise

Other

TIME

	begin	end	duration		begin	end	duration
1				3			
2				4			

LOCATION

SEVERITY

1	2	3	4	5	6	7	8	9	10

MILD   SEVERE

TRIGGERS

coffee	insomnia	eye strain	smell
alcohol	stress	sickness	
medication	bright light	travel	
food	pc/tv screen	motion	
weather	reading	anxiety	
allergies	noise	pms	

RELIEF MEASURES

medication

sleep/rest

exercise

Other

<table>
<tr><td></td><td colspan="3">DATE</td><td colspan="4"></td></tr>
</table>

DATE

TIME

	begin	end	duration		begin	end	duration
1				3			
2				4			

LOCATION

tension	gca	cluster	sinus	migraine	neck

SEVERITY

1	2	3	4	5	6	7	8	9	10

MILD   SEVERE

TRIGGERS

☐ coffee	☐ insomnia	☐ eye strain	☐ smell
☐ alcohol	☐ stress	☐ sickness	☐
☐ medication	☐ bright light	☐ travel	☐
☐ food	☐ pc/tv screen	☐ motion	☐
☐ weather	☐ reading	☐ anxiety	☐
☐ allergies	☐ noise	☐ pms	☐

RELIEF MEASURES

medication

sleep/rest

exercise

Other

<table>
<tr><td></td><td colspan="3">DATE</td><td></td></tr>
</table>

TIME

	begin	end	duration		begin	end	duration
1				3			
2				4			

LOCATION

tension	gca	cluster	sinus	migraine	neck
□□□□	□□□□	□□□□	□□□□	□□□□	□□□□

SEVERITY

1	2	3	4	5	6	7	8	9	10

MILD — SEVERE

TRIGGERS

□ coffee	□ insomnia	□ eye strain	□ smell
□ alcohol	□ stress	□ sickness	□
□ medication	□ bright light	□ travel	□
□ food	□ pc/tv screen	□ motion	□
□ weather	□ reading	□ anxiety	□
□ allergies	□ noise	□ pms	□

RELIEF MEASURES

medication	
sleep/rest	
exercise	
Other	

TIME

	begin	end	duration		begin	end	duration
1				3			
2				4			

LOCATION

tension	gca	cluster	sinus	migraine	neck

SEVERITY

1	2	3	4	5	6	7	8	9	10

MILD — SEVERE

TRIGGERS

☐ coffee	☐ insomnia	☐ eye strain	☐ smell
☐ alcohol	☐ stress	☐ sickness	☐
☐ medication	☐ bright light	☐ travel	☐
☐ food	☐ pc/tv screen	☐ motion	☐
☐ weather	☐ reading	☐ anxiety	☐
☐ allergies	☐ noise	☐ pms	☐

RELIEF MEASURES

medication

sleep/rest

exercise

Other

TIME

	begin	end	duration		begin	end	duration
1				3			
2				4			

LOCATION

tension | gca | cluster | sinus | migraine | neck

SEVERITY

1	2	3	4	5	6	7	8	9	10

MILD | SEVERE

TRIGGERS

☐ coffee	☐ insomnia	☐ eye strain	☐ smell
☐ alcohol	☐ stress	☐ sickness	☐
☐ medication	☐ bright light	☐ travel	☐
☐ food	☐ pc/tv screen	☐ motion	☐
☐ weather	☐ reading	☐ anxiety	☐
☐ allergies	☐ noise	☐ pms	☐

RELIEF MEASURES

medication

sleep/rest

exercise

Other

<table>
<tr><td colspan="7" align="center">DATE</td></tr>
</table>

TIME

	begin	end	duration		begin	end	duration
1				3			
2				4			

LOCATION

tension	gca	cluster	sinus	migraine	neck

SEVERITY

1	2	3	4	5	6	7	8	9	10

MILD   SEVERE

TRIGGERS

☐ coffee	☐ insomnia	☐ eye strain	☐ smell
☐ alcohol	☐ stress	☐ sickness	☐
☐ medication	☐ bright light	☐ travel	☐
☐ food	☐ pc/tv screen	☐ motion	☐
☐ weather	☐ reading	☐ anxiety	☐
☐ allergies	☐ noise	☐ pms	☐

RELIEF MEASURES

medication	
sleep/rest	
exercise	
Other	

DATE	

TIME

	begin	end	duration		begin	end	duration
1				3			
2				4			

LOCATION

tension	gca	cluster	sinus	migraine	neck

SEVERITY

1	2	3	4	5	6	7	8	9	10

MILD · SEVERE

TRIGGERS

☐ coffee	☐ insomnia	☐ eye strain	☐ smell
☐ alcohol	☐ stress	☐ sickness	☐
☐ medication	☐ bright light	☐ travel	☐
☐ food	☐ pc/tv screen	☐ motion	☐
☐ weather	☐ reading	☐ anxiety	☐
☐ allergies	☐ noise	☐ pms	☐

RELIEF MEASURES

medication	
sleep/rest	
exercise	
Other	

<table>
<tr><td colspan="7" style="text-align:center">DATE</td></tr>
</table>

TIME

	begin	end	duration		begin	end	duration
1				3			
2				4			

LOCATION

tension	gca	cluster	sinus	migraine	neck

SEVERITY

1	2	3	4	5	6	7	8	9	10

MILD   SEVERE

TRIGGERS

☐ coffee	☐ insomnia	☐ eye strain	☐ smell
☐ alcohol	☐ stress	☐ sickness	☐
☐ medication	☐ bright light	☐ travel	☐
☐ food	☐ pc/tv screen	☐ motion	☐
☐ weather	☐ reading	☐ anxiety	☐
☐ allergies	☐ noise	☐ pms	☐

RELIEF MEASURES

medication

sleep/rest

exercise

Other

<table>
<tr><td></td><td>**DATE**</td><td></td></tr>
</table>

TIME

	begin	end	duration		begin	end	duration
1				3			
2				4			

LOCATION

tension	gca	cluster	sinus	migraine	neck
□□□□	□□□□	□□□□	□□□□	□□□□	□□□□

SEVERITY

1	2	3	4	5	6	7	8	9	10

MILD — SEVERE

TRIGGERS

☐ coffee	☐ insomnia	☐ eye strain	☐ smell
☐ alcohol	☐ stress	☐ sickness	☐
☐ medication	☐ bright light	☐ travel	☐
☐ food	☐ pc/tv screen	☐ motion	☐
☐ weather	☐ reading	☐ anxiety	☐
☐ allergies	☐ noise	☐ pms	☐

RELIEF MEASURES

medication

sleep/rest

exercise

Other

<table>
<tr><td></td><td></td><td></td><td></td><td style="text-align:center">DATE</td><td></td><td></td><td></td></tr>
</table>

TIME

	begin	end	duration		begin	end	duration
1				3			
2				4			

LOCATION

tension	gca	cluster	sinus	migraine	neck

SEVERITY

1	2	3	4	5	6	7	8	9	10

MILD   SEVERE

TRIGGERS

☐ coffee	☐ insomnia	☐ eye strain	☐ smell
☐ alcohol	☐ stress	☐ sickness	☐
☐ medication	☐ bright light	☐ travel	☐
☐ food	☐ pc/tv screen	☐ motion	☐
☐ weather	☐ reading	☐ anxiety	☐
☐ allergies	☐ noise	☐ pms	☐

RELIEF MEASURES

medication

sleep/rest

exercise

Other

<table>
<tr><td colspan="7" align="center">DATE</td></tr>
</table>

TIME

	begin	end	duration		begin	end	duration
1				3			
2				4			

LOCATION

tension	gca	cluster	sinus	migraine	neck

SEVERITY

1	2	3	4	5	6	7	8	9	10

MILD   SEVERE

TRIGGERS

☐ coffee	☐ insomnia	☐ eye strain	☐ smell
☐ alcohol	☐ stress	☐ sickness	☐
☐ medication	☐ bright light	☐ travel	☐
☐ food	☐ pc/tv screen	☐ motion	☐
☐ weather	☐ reading	☐ anxiety	☐
☐ allergies	☐ noise	☐ pms	☐

RELIEF MEASURES

medication

sleep/rest

exercise

Other

<table>
<tr><td></td><td>DATE</td><td></td></tr>
</table>

TIME

	begin	end	duration		begin	end	duration
1				3			
2				4			

LOCATION

tension	gca	cluster	sinus	migraine	neck

SEVERITY

1	2	3	4	5	6	7	8	9	10

MILD   SEVERE

TRIGGERS

☐ coffee	☐ insomnia	☐ eye strain	☐ smell
☐ alcohol	☐ stress	☐ sickness	☐
☐ medication	☐ bright light	☐ travel	☐
☐ food	☐ pc/tv screen	☐ motion	☐
☐ weather	☐ reading	☐ anxiety	☐
☐ allergies	☐ noise	☐ pms	☐

RELIEF MEASURES

medication	
sleep/rest	
exercise	
Other	

<table>
<tr><td colspan="7" align="center">DATE</td></tr>
</table>

<table>
<tr><td colspan="7" align="center">TIME</td></tr>
<tr><td></td><td>begin</td><td>end</td><td>duration</td><td>begin</td><td>end</td><td>duration</td></tr>
<tr><td>1</td><td></td><td></td><td></td><td>3</td><td></td><td></td></tr>
<tr><td>2</td><td></td><td></td><td></td><td>4</td><td></td><td></td></tr>
</table>

LOCATION

tension	gca	cluster	sinus	migraine	neck

SEVERITY

1	2	3	4	5	6	7	8	9	10

MILD   SEVERE

TRIGGERS

☐ coffee	☐ insomnia	☐ eye strain	☐ smell
☐ alcohol	☐ stress	☐ sickness	☐
☐ medication	☐ bright light	☐ travel	☐
☐ food	☐ pc/tv screen	☐ motion	☐
☐ weather	☐ reading	☐ anxiety	☐
☐ allergies	☐ noise	☐ pms	☐

RELIEF MEASURES

medication	
sleep/rest	
exercise	
Other	

<table>
<tr><td></td><td></td><td></td><td></td><td style="background:gray;color:white">DATE</td><td></td><td></td></tr>
</table>

TIME

	begin	end	duration		begin	end	duration
1				3			
2				4			

LOCATION

tension	gca	cluster	sinus	migraine	neck

SEVERITY

1	2	3	4	5	6	7	8	9	10

MILD   SEVERE

TRIGGERS

☐ coffee	☐ insomnia	☐ eye strain	☐ smell
☐ alcohol	☐ stress	☐ sickness	☐
☐ medication	☐ bright light	☐ travel	☐
☐ food	☐ pc/tv screen	☐ motion	☐
☐ weather	☐ reading	☐ anxiety	☐
☐ allergies	☐ noise	☐ pms	☐

RELIEF MEASURES

medication

sleep/rest

exercise

Other

	begin	end	duration		begin	end	duration
1				3			
2				4			

tension	gca	cluster	sinus	migraine	neck

1	2	3	4	5	6	7	8	9	10

MILD   SEVERE

- ☐ coffee
- ☐ alcohol
- ☐ medication
- ☐ food
- ☐ weather
- ☐ allergies
- ☐ insomnia
- ☐ stress
- ☐ bright light
- ☐ pc/tv screen
- ☐ reading
- ☐ noise
- ☐ eye strain
- ☐ sickness
- ☐ travel
- ☐ motion
- ☐ anxiety
- ☐ pms
- ☐ smell

medication

sleep/rest

exercise

Other

<table>
<tr><td></td><td>DATE</td><td></td></tr>
</table>

TIME

	begin	end	duration		begin	end	duration
1				3			
2				4			

LOCATION

tension	gca	cluster	sinus	migraine	neck

SEVERITY

1	2	3	4	5	6	7	8	9	10

MILD   SEVERE

TRIGGERS

☐ coffee	☐ insomnia	☐ eye strain	☐ smell
☐ alcohol	☐ stress	☐ sickness	☐
☐ medication	☐ bright light	☐ travel	☐
☐ food	☐ pc/tv screen	☐ motion	☐
☐ weather	☐ reading	☐ anxiety	☐
☐ allergies	☐ noise	☐ pms	☐

RELIEF MEASURES

medication

sleep/rest

exercise

Other

<table>
<tr><td></td><td>DATE</td><td></td></tr>
</table>

TIME

	begin	end	duration		begin	end	duration
1				3			
2				4			

LOCATION

tension	gca	cluster	sinus	migraine	neck

SEVERITY

1	2	3	4	5	6	7	8	9	10

MILD   SEVERE

TRIGGERS

☐ coffee	☐ insomnia	☐ eye strain	☐ smell
☐ alcohol	☐ stress	☐ sickness	☐
☐ medication	☐ bright light	☐ travel	☐
☐ food	☐ pc/tv screen	☐ motion	☐
☐ weather	☐ reading	☐ anxiety	☐
☐ allergies	☐ noise	☐ pms	☐

RELIEF MEASURES

medication

sleep/rest

exercise

Other

<table>
<tr><td></td><td style="text-align:center">DATE</td><td></td></tr>
</table>

TIME

	begin	end	duration		begin	end	duration
1				3			
2				4			

LOCATION

tension	gca	cluster	sinus	migraine	neck

SEVERITY

1	2	3	4	5	6	7	8	9	10

MILD | SEVERE

TRIGGERS

☐ coffee	☐ insomnia	☐ eye strain	☐ smell
☐ alcohol	☐ stress	☐ sickness	☐
☐ medication	☐ bright light	☐ travel	☐
☐ food	☐ pc/tv screen	☐ motion	☐
☐ weather	☐ reading	☐ anxiety	☐
☐ allergies	☐ noise	☐ pms	☐

RELIEF MEASURES

medication	
sleep/rest	
exercise	
Other	

<table>
<tr><td></td><td>DATE</td><td></td></tr>
</table>

TIME

	begin	end	duration		begin	end	duration
1				3			
2				4			

LOCATION

tension	gca	cluster	sinus	migraine	neck

SEVERITY

1	2	3	4	5	6	7	8	9	10

MILD   SEVERE

TRIGGERS

☐ coffee	☐ insomnia	☐ eye strain	☐ smell
☐ alcohol	☐ stress	☐ sickness	☐
☐ medication	☐ bright light	☐ travel	☐
☐ food	☐ pc/tv screen	☐ motion	☐
☐ weather	☐ reading	☐ anxiety	☐
☐ allergies	☐ noise	☐ pms	☐

RELIEF MEASURES

medication	
sleep/rest	
exercise	
Other	

<table>
<tr><td colspan="7" align="center">DATE</td></tr>
</table>

TIME

	begin	end	duration		begin	end	duration
1				3			
2				4			

LOCATION

tension	gca	cluster	sinus	migraine	neck

SEVERITY

1	2	3	4	5	6	7	8	9	10

MILD   SEVERE

TRIGGERS

- [ ] coffee
- [ ] alcohol
- [ ] medication
- [ ] food
- [ ] weather
- [ ] allergies
- [ ] insomnia
- [ ] stress
- [ ] bright light
- [ ] pc/tv screen
- [ ] reading
- [ ] noise
- [ ] eye strain
- [ ] sickness
- [ ] travel
- [ ] motion
- [ ] anxiety
- [ ] pms
- [ ] smell

RELIEF MEASURES

medication

sleep/rest

exercise

Other

<table>
<tr><td></td><td style="text-align:center">DATE</td><td></td></tr>
</table>

TIME

	begin	end	duration		begin	end	duration
1				3			
2				4			

LOCATION

tension	gca	cluster	sinus	migraine	neck

SEVERITY

1	2	3	4	5	6	7	8	9	10

MILD   SEVERE

TRIGGERS

☐ coffee	☐ insomnia	☐ eye strain	☐ smell
☐ alcohol	☐ stress	☐ sickness	☐
☐ medication	☐ bright light	☐ travel	☐
☐ food	☐ pc/tv screen	☐ motion	☐
☐ weather	☐ reading	☐ anxiety	☐
☐ allergies	☐ noise	☐ pms	☐

RELIEF MEASURES

medication

sleep/rest

exercise

Other

<table>
<tr><td></td><td colspan="6">DATE</td></tr>
</table>

TIME

	begin	end	duration		begin	end	duration
1				3			
2				4			

LOCATION

tension	gca	cluster	sinus	migraine	neck

SEVERITY

1	2	3	4	5	6	7	8	9	10

MILD   SEVERE

TRIGGERS

☐ coffee	☐ insomnia	☐ eye strain	☐ smell
☐ alcohol	☐ stress	☐ sickness	☐
☐ medication	☐ bright light	☐ travel	☐
☐ food	☐ pc/tv screen	☐ motion	☐
☐ weather	☐ reading	☐ anxiety	☐
☐ allergies	☐ noise	☐ pms	☐

RELIEF MEASURES

medication

sleep/rest

exercise

Other

<table>
<tr><td></td><td>DATE</td><td></td></tr>
</table>

TIME

	begin	end	duration		begin	end	duration
1				3			
2				4			

LOCATION

tension	gca	cluster	sinus	migraine	neck

SEVERITY

1	2	3	4	5	6	7	8	9	10

MILD · SEVERE

TRIGGERS

☐ coffee	☐ insomnia	☐ eye strain	☐ smell
☐ alcohol	☐ stress	☐ sickness	☐
☐ medication	☐ bright light	☐ travel	☐
☐ food	☐ pc/tv screen	☐ motion	☐
☐ weather	☐ reading	☐ anxiety	☐
☐ allergies	☐ noise	☐ pms	☐

RELIEF MEASURES

medication

sleep/rest

exercise

Other

<table>
<tr><td></td><td></td><td></td><td></td><td>DATE</td><td></td></tr>
</table>

TIME

	begin	end	duration		begin	end	duration
1				3			
2				4			

LOCATION

tension	gca	cluster	sinus	migraine	neck

SEVERITY

1	2	3	4	5	6	7	8	9	10

MILD   SEVERE

TRIGGERS

☐ coffee	☐ insomnia	☐ eye strain	☐ smell
☐ alcohol	☐ stress	☐ sickness	☐
☐ medication	☐ bright light	☐ travel	☐
☐ food	☐ pc/tv screen	☐ motion	☐
☐ weather	☐ reading	☐ anxiety	☐
☐ allergies	☐ noise	☐ pms	☐

RELIEF MEASURES

medication	
sleep/rest	
exercise	
Other	

<table>
<tr><td></td><td>**DATE**</td><td></td></tr>
</table>

TIME

	begin	end	duration		begin	end	duration
1				3			
2				4			

LOCATION

tension	gca	cluster	sinus	migraine	neck

SEVERITY

1	2	3	4	5	6	7	8	9	10

MILD   SEVERE

TRIGGERS

☐ coffee	☐ insomnia	☐ eye strain	☐ smell
☐ alcohol	☐ stress	☐ sickness	☐
☐ medication	☐ bright light	☐ travel	☐
☐ food	☐ pc/tv screen	☐ motion	☐
☐ weather	☐ reading	☐ anxiety	☐
☐ allergies	☐ noise	☐ pms	☐

RELIEF MEASURES

medication	
sleep/rest	
exercise	
Other	

<table>
<tr><td></td><td></td><td></td><td></td><td></td><td>DATE</td><td></td><td></td></tr>
</table>

TIME

	begin	end	duration		begin	end	duration
1				3			
2				4			

LOCATION

tension	gca	cluster	sinus	migraine	neck

SEVERITY

1	2	3	4	5	6	7	8	9	10

MILD   SEVERE

TRIGGERS

☐ coffee	☐ insomnia	☐ eye strain	☐ smell
☐ alcohol	☐ stress	☐ sickness	☐
☐ medication	☐ bright light	☐ travel	☐
☐ food	☐ pc/tv screen	☐ motion	☐
☐ weather	☐ reading	☐ anxiety	☐
☐ allergies	☐ noise	☐ pms	☐

RELIEF MEASURES

medication

sleep/rest

exercise

Other

TIME

	begin	end	duration		begin	end	duration
1				3			
2				4			

LOCATION

tension	gca	cluster	sinus	migraine	neck

SEVERITY

1	2	3	4	5	6	7	8	9	10

MILD — SEVERE

TRIGGERS

☐ coffee	☐ insomnia	☐ eye strain	☐ smell
☐ alcohol	☐ stress	☐ sickness	☐
☐ medication	☐ bright light	☐ travel	☐
☐ food	☐ pc/tv screen	☐ motion	☐
☐ weather	☐ reading	☐ anxiety	☐
☐ allergies	☐ noise	☐ pms	☐

RELIEF MEASURES

medication

sleep/rest

exercise

Other

TIME

	begin	end	duration		begin	end	duration
1				3			
2				4			

LOCATION

tension	gca	cluster	sinus	migraine	neck

SEVERITY

1	2	3	4	5	6	7	8	9	10

MILD · SEVERE

TRIGGERS

- [ ] coffee
- [ ] alcohol
- [ ] medication
- [ ] food
- [ ] weather
- [ ] allergies
- [ ] insomnia
- [ ] stress
- [ ] bright light
- [ ] pc/tv screen
- [ ] reading
- [ ] noise
- [ ] eye strain
- [ ] sickness
- [ ] travel
- [ ] motion
- [ ] anxiety
- [ ] pms
- [ ] smell

RELIEF MEASURES

medication

sleep/rest

exercise

Other

<table><tr><td></td><td>DATE</td><td></td></tr></table>

TIME

	begin	end	duration		begin	end	duration
1				3			
2				4			

LOCATION

tension	gca	cluster	sinus	migraine	neck

SEVERITY

1	2	3	4	5	6	7	8	9	10

MILD   SEVERE

TRIGGERS

☐ coffee	☐ insomnia	☐ eye strain	☐ smell
☐ alcohol	☐ stress	☐ sickness	☐
☐ medication	☐ bright light	☐ travel	☐
☐ food	☐ pc/tv screen	☐ motion	☐
☐ weather	☐ reading	☐ anxiety	☐
☐ allergies	☐ noise	☐ pms	☐

RELIEF MEASURES

medication	
sleep/rest	
exercise	
Other	

<table>
<tr><td></td><td style="background:gray">DATE</td><td></td></tr>
</table>

TIME

	begin	end	duration		begin	end	duration
1				3			
2				4			

LOCATION

tension	gca	cluster	sinus	migraine	neck

SEVERITY

1	2	3	4	5	6	7	8	9	10

MILD   SEVERE

TRIGGERS

☐ coffee	☐ insomnia	☐ eye strain	☐ smell
☐ alcohol	☐ stress	☐ sickness	☐
☐ medication	☐ bright light	☐ travel	☐
☐ food	☐ pc/tv screen	☐ motion	☐
☐ weather	☐ reading	☐ anxiety	☐
☐ allergies	☐ noise	☐ pms	☐

RELIEF MEASURES

medication	
sleep/rest	
exercise	
Other	

TIME

	begin	end	duration		begin	end	duration
1				3			
2				4			

LOCATION

tension	gca	cluster	sinus	migraine	neck

SEVERITY

1	2	3	4	5	6	7	8	9	10

MILD   SEVERE

TRIGGERS

☐ coffee	☐ insomnia	☐ eye strain	☐ smell
☐ alcohol	☐ stress	☐ sickness	☐
☐ medication	☐ bright light	☐ travel	☐
☐ food	☐ pc/tv screen	☐ motion	☐
☐ weather	☐ reading	☐ anxiety	☐
☐ allergies	☐ noise	☐ pms	☐

RELIEF MEASURES

medication

sleep/rest

exercise

Other

<table>
<tr><td></td><td>DATE</td><td></td></tr>
</table>

TIME

	begin	end	duration		begin	end	duration
1				3			
2				4			

LOCATION

tension	gca	cluster	sinus	migraine	neck

SEVERITY

1	2	3	4	5	6	7	8	9	10

MILD — SEVERE

TRIGGERS

☐ coffee	☐ insomnia	☐ eye strain	☐ smell
☐ alcohol	☐ stress	☐ sickness	☐
☐ medication	☐ bright light	☐ travel	☐
☐ food	☐ pc/tv screen	☐ motion	☐
☐ weather	☐ reading	☐ anxiety	☐
☐ allergies	☐ noise	☐ pms	☐

RELIEF MEASURES

medication

sleep/rest

exercise

Other

DATE	

TIME

	begin	end	duration		begin	end	duration
1				3			
2				4			

LOCATION

tension	gca	cluster	sinus	migraine	neck

SEVERITY

1	2	3	4	5	6	7	8	9	10

MILD — SEVERE

TRIGGERS

☐ coffee	☐ insomnia	☐ eye strain	☐ smell
☐ alcohol	☐ stress	☐ sickness	☐
☐ medication	☐ bright light	☐ travel	☐
☐ food	☐ pc/tv screen	☐ motion	☐
☐ weather	☐ reading	☐ anxiety	☐
☐ allergies	☐ noise	☐ pms	☐

RELIEF MEASURES

medication	
sleep/rest	
exercise	
Other	

DATE	

TIME

	begin	end	duration		begin	end	duration
1				3			
2				4			

LOCATION

tension	gca	cluster	sinus	migraine	neck
□□□□	□□□□	□□□□	□□□□	□□□□	□□□□

SEVERITY

1	2	3	4	5	6	7	8	9	10

MILD — SEVERE

TRIGGERS

☐ coffee	☐ insomnia	☐ eye strain	☐ smell
☐ alcohol	☐ stress	☐ sickness	☐
☐ medication	☐ bright light	☐ travel	☐
☐ food	☐ pc/tv screen	☐ motion	☐
☐ weather	☐ reading	☐ anxiety	☐
☐ allergies	☐ noise	☐ pms	☐

RELIEF MEASURES

medication

sleep/rest

exercise

Other

DATE

TIME

	begin	end	duration		begin	end	duration
1				3			
2				4			

LOCATION

tension	gca	cluster	sinus	migraine	neck

SEVERITY

1	2	3	4	5	6	7	8	9	10

MILD   SEVERE

TRIGGERS

- ☐ coffee
- ☐ alcohol
- ☐ medication
- ☐ food
- ☐ weather
- ☐ allergies
- ☐ insomnia
- ☐ stress
- ☐ bright light
- ☐ pc/tv screen
- ☐ reading
- ☐ noise
- ☐ eye strain
- ☐ sickness
- ☐ travel
- ☐ motion
- ☐ anxiety
- ☐ pms
- ☐ smell

RELIEF MEASURES

medication

sleep/rest

exercise

Other

<table>
<tr><td></td><td colspan="6" align="center">DATE</td></tr>
</table>

TIME

	begin	end	duration		begin	end	duration
1				3			
2				4			

LOCATION

tension	gca	cluster	sinus	migraine	neck

SEVERITY

1	2	3	4	5	6	7	8	9	10

MILD   SEVERE

TRIGGERS

coffee	insomnia	eye strain	smell
alcohol	stress	sickness	
medication	bright light	travel	
food	pc/tv screen	motion	
weather	reading	anxiety	
allergies	noise	pms	

RELIEF MEASURES

medication	
sleep/rest	
exercise	
Other	

<table>
<tr><td></td><td>DATE</td><td></td></tr>
</table>

TIME

	begin	end	duration		begin	end	duration
1				3			
2				4			

LOCATION

tension	gca	cluster	sinus	migraine	neck

SEVERITY

1	2	3	4	5	6	7	8	9	10

MILD   SEVERE

TRIGGERS

☐ coffee	☐ insomnia	☐ eye strain	☐ smell
☐ alcohol	☐ stress	☐ sickness	☐
☐ medication	☐ bright light	☐ travel	☐
☐ food	☐ pc/tv screen	☐ motion	☐
☐ weather	☐ reading	☐ anxiety	☐
☐ allergies	☐ noise	☐ pms	☐

RELIEF MEASURES

medication

sleep/rest

exercise

Other

<table>
<tr><td></td><td colspan="6">DATE</td></tr>
</table>

TIME

	begin	end	duration		begin	end	duration
1				3			
2				4			

LOCATION

tension	gca	cluster	sinus	migraine	neck

SEVERITY

1	2	3	4	5	6	7	8	9	10

MILD · SEVERE

TRIGGERS

☐ coffee	☐ insomnia	☐ eye strain	☐ smell
☐ alcohol	☐ stress	☐ sickness	☐
☐ medication	☐ bright light	☐ travel	☐
☐ food	☐ pc/tv screen	☐ motion	☐
☐ weather	☐ reading	☐ anxiety	☐
☐ allergies	☐ noise	☐ pms	☐

RELIEF MEASURES

medication	
sleep/rest	
exercise	
Other	

<table><tr><td></td><td>DATE</td><td></td></tr></table>

TIME

	begin	end	duration		begin	end	duration
1				3			
2				4			

LOCATION

tension	gca	cluster	sinus	migraine	neck

SEVERITY

1	2	3	4	5	6	7	8	9	10

MILD — SEVERE

TRIGGERS

☐ coffee	☐ insomnia	☐ eye strain	☐ smell
☐ alcohol	☐ stress	☐ sickness	☐
☐ medication	☐ bright light	☐ travel	☐
☐ food	☐ pc/tv screen	☐ motion	☐
☐ weather	☐ reading	☐ anxiety	☐
☐ allergies	☐ noise	☐ pms	☐

RELIEF MEASURES

medication

sleep/rest

exercise

Other

<table>
<tr><td></td><td>DATE</td><td></td></tr>
</table>

TIME

	begin	end	duration		begin	end	duration
1				3			
2				4			

LOCATION

tension	gca	cluster	sinus	migraine	neck

SEVERITY

1	2	3	4	5	6	7	8	9	10

MILD   SEVERE

TRIGGERS

☐ coffee	☐ insomnia	☐ eye strain	☐ smell
☐ alcohol	☐ stress	☐ sickness	☐
☐ medication	☐ bright light	☐ travel	☐
☐ food	☐ pc/tv screen	☐ motion	☐
☐ weather	☐ reading	☐ anxiety	☐
☐ allergies	☐ noise	☐ pms	☐

RELIEF MEASURES

medication

sleep/rest

exercise

Other

www.ingramcontent.com/pod-product-compliance
Lightning Source LLC
Chambersburg PA
CBHW070746250726
48662CB00004B/1662